Copyright © 2022 by Monica Dimitrios

Table of Contents

ALKALINE

Alkaline diet describes a group of loosely related diets based on the misconception that different types of food can have an effect on the pH balance of the body. It originated from the acid ash hypothesis, which primarily related to osteoporosis research.

The alkaline diet, also called the alkaline-ash diet or alkaline-acid diet, was made popular by its celebrity followers. Big names like Victoria Beckham, Kate Hudson, and Tom Brady have said that they've tried the diet with positive results.

ALKALINE RECIPES

1. Breaded Brussels Sprouts

Prep Time: 25 mins

Total Time: 37 mins

Servings: 8

Ingredients

- 1 ½ pounds Brussels sprouts
- 1 teaspoon salt
- 4 tablespoons butter, melted
- 4 tablespoons grated Parmesan cheese
- 4 tablespoons dried bread crumbs
- ¼ teaspoon garlic powder
- ¼ teaspoon ground black pepper
- ¼ teaspoon seasoning salt

Directions

1. Wash and trim Brussels sprouts. Cut an "X" about 1/8 inch deep in the stem of the sprouts (this helps cook the sprouts more evenly and quickly).
2. In a medium-size pot, cover Brussels sprouts with water; add 1 teaspoon salt and bring to boil. Cover and simmer for 6 minutes or until tender; drain. Be careful not to overcook sprouts.

3. Place sprouts in a small casserole dish. Sprinkle 2 tablespoons of melted butter over the sprouts and mix well to coat.
4. Combine Parmesan cheese, dried bread crumbs, garlic powder, black pepper, seasoning salt, and remaining butter and mix well; sprinkle mixture over sprouts.
5. Heat sprouts under broiler (about 4 inches away from heat) for about 5 minutes or until crumb mixture is lightly browned. Serve hot.

Prep Time 10 mins

Total Time: 1 hr 55 mins

Servings: 12

Ingredients

- 2 (.25 ounce) packages active dry yeast
- 1 ½ cups warm water (110 degrees F/45 degrees C)
- ½ cup shortening, melted and cooled slightly
- ½ cup white sugar
- 2 teaspoons salt
- 4 ½ cups all-purpose flour
- 2 tablespoons butter, melted

Directions

1. In a large bowl, dissolve yeast in warm water. Let stand until creamy, about 10 minutes.
2. Stir in shortening, sugar, salt and 2 cups flour; beat well. Stir in the remaining flour, 1/2 cup at a time, beating well after each addition. Scrape sides of bowl, cover and let rise until doubled in size, about 1 hour.

3. Grease 12 muffin cups. Spoon in batter until cups are half full. Let rise in warm place until batter reaches top of the cup, about 20 to 30 minutes.
4. Preheat oven to 425 degrees F (220 degrees C).
5. Bake in preheated oven for 10 to 15 minutes. Remove from pans and brush tops with melted butter.

3. Lentil and Eggplant Moussaka

Prep Time: 35 mins

Total Time: 1 hr 50 mins

Servings: 4

Ingredients

- 1 ½ pounds eggplant, cut into 1/4-inch slices
- 1 pound tomatoes, stems removed
- 2 tablespoons olive oil
- 2 medium onions, minced
- 3 cloves garlic, minced
- ½ cup beluga lentils
- 2 tablespoons tomato paste
- 1 ½ cups vegetable broth
- 1 ½ pounds zucchini, chopped
- 1 tablespoon dried savory
- 1 teaspoon ground cinnamon
- 1 teaspoon ground cumin
- ¾ cup crumbled feta cheese
- 1 ¼ cups plain Greek yogurt
- 4 large eggs

Directions

1. Bring a large pot of salted water to a boil. Blanch eggplant slices in the boiling water for 1 minute. Rinse slices under cold water, then drain on paper towels.
2. Blanch tomatoes in the boiling water for 1 minute. Rinse in cold water, then remove skins. Cut tomatoes into quarters and remove and discard the cores. Chop tomatoes coarsely.
3. Heat olive oil in a saucepan over medium heat. Add onions and garlic and sauté until translucent, about 5 minutes. Add lentils and tomato paste; sauté briefly. Add vegetable broth, cover, and bring to a boil. Reduce heat to low and simmer for 15 minutes.
4. Add chopped tomatoes, zucchini, savory, cinnamon, and cumin. Cover, increase heat, and bring to a boil. Reduce heat to low and simmer for 10 more minutes.
5. Preheat the oven to 425 degrees F (220 degrees C).
6. Pour 1/2 of the lentil mixture into the bottom of a large oven-proof dish. Cover with 1/2 of the eggplant slices. Pour remaining lentil mixture over top and cover with remaining eggplant slices.
7. Mash feta cheese with a fork; mix with yogurt and eggs. Season with salt and pepper. Spread over the eggplant layer.

8. Bake in the center of the preheated oven until
   golden brown, about 25 minutes.

4. Strawberry Yogurt Cake

Prep Time: 20 mins

Total Time: 2 hrs 20 mins

Servings: 12

Ingredients

- 1 (18.25 ounce) box Betty Crocker SuperMoist white cake mix
- ¾ cup water
- ⅓ cup vegetable oil
- 3 large egg whites egg whites
- 1 (6 ounce) container Yoplait Original 99% Fat Free strawberry yogurt
- 1 (12 ounce) container Betty Crocker Whipped vanilla frosting
- 4 cups strawberries

Directions

1. Heat oven to 350 degrees F (325 degrees F for dark or nonstick pans). Generously grease and lightly flour bottoms and sides of two 8-inch or 9-inch round pans, or spray with baking spray with flour.
2. In large bowl, beat cake mix, water, oil, egg whites and yogurt with electric mixer on low speed 30

seconds; beat on medium speed 2 minutes (batter will be lumpy). Pour into pans.

3. Bake 8-inch rounds 27 to 32 minutes, 9-inch rounds 25 to 30 minutes, or until toothpick inserted in center comes out clean. Cool 10 minutes. Run knife around sides of pans to loosen cakes; remove from pans to cooling rack. Cool completely, about 1 hour.

4. Spread 1/3 cup frosting over 1 cake layer to within 1/4 inch of edge. Cut about 10 strawberries into 1/4-inch slices; arrange on frosted layer. Top with second layer. Frost side and top of cake with remaining frosting. Cut remaining strawberries in half; arrange on top of cake. Store loosely covered in refrigerator.

5. Fruitcake Cookies II

Servings: 48

Ingredients

- 4 cups all-purpose flour
- 1 teaspoon baking soda
- 1 teaspoon salt
- 1 cup shortening
- 2 cups packed brown sugar
- 2 eggs
- ⅔ cup milk
- 1 cup chopped pecans
- 2 cups dates, pitted and chopped
- 1 cup candied cherries, quartered
- 1 cup candied mixed citrus peel
- ½ cup red and green candied cherries, halved

Directions

1. Sift the flour, measure and sift it again with the baking soda and salt.
2. Cream the shortening add the sugar and eggs. Beat until light and fluffy. Add the milk and flour mixture, mixing well. Stir in the nuts, dates, cherries and candied peel. Cover and chill dough for several hours.
3. Preheat oven to 350 degrees F (175 degrees C).

4. Drop chilled dough by teaspoons, 2 inches apart, onto lightly greased baking sheets. Top each cookie with a half of a candied cherry. Bake at 350 degrees F (175 degrees C) for 8 to 10 minutes.

6. Buffalo Cheesy Chicken Lasagna

Prep Time: 15 mins

Total Time: 1 hr 50 mins

Servings: 10

Ingredients

- 1 pound skinless, boneless chicken breast - cooked and diced
- 4 cups spaghetti sauce
- 2 tablespoons hot sauce
- 2 tablespoons apple cider vinegar
- 1 ½ cups water
- 1 teaspoon garlic powder
- 1 small onion, chopped
- 1 small green bell pepper, chopped
- 1 (6 ounce) can mushrooms, drained
- 1 egg, beaten
- 1 (15 ounce) container ricotta cheese
- 12 uncooked lasagna noodles
- 2 cups shredded mozzarella cheese
- ¾ cup crumbled blue cheese

Directions

1. Preheat oven to 350 degrees F (175 degrees C).
   Lightly grease a lasagna pan.
2. In a large bowl combine the chicken, spaghetti
   sauce, hot sauce, vinegar, water, garlic powder,
   onion, bell pepper and mushrooms; mix well and
   set aside. In a medium bowl, mix together the egg
   beat and ricotta cheese.
3. Spread 1 cup of the chicken/spaghetti mixture in
   the bottom of the prepared pan. Layer with
   lasagna noodles, then another 1 1/2 cups of the
   chicken mixture. Spread 1/2 of the ricotta/egg
   mixture over all, then top with 1/2 of the
   mozzarella cheese. Add another layer of noodles, 1
   1/2 cups chicken mixture, remaining ricotta
   mixture and remaining mozzarella. Top with one
   last layer of noodles and remaining chicken
   mixture.
4. Cover pan and bake at 350 degrees F (175 degrees
   C) for 70 minutes. Remove cover, sprinkle with
   crumbled blue cheese and bake uncovered for
   another 5 minutes.
5. Remove from oven, cover and let stand for about
   15 to 20 minutes before serving.

Prep Time: 25 mins

Total Time: 55 mins

Servings: 6

Ingredients

- 1 tablespoon clarified butter
- 1 ⅓ pounds quinces - peeled, cored, and cut into wedges
- ½ cup all-purpose flour
- 1 tablespoon white sugar
- 1 pinch salt
- ½ cup dark beer
- 1 dash vanilla extract
- 2 teaspoons finely grated fresh lemon zest
- 3 tablespoons coconut oil, or as needed
- 3 tablespoons demerara sugar

Directions

1. Heat the clarified butter in a skillet over low heat, and place the quince wedges into the pan. Cover, then gently cook the quince wedges until softened, about 15 minutes. Remove from heat and set aside.

2. Mix the flour, white sugar, and salt in a bowl. In a separate bowl, mix the beer with the vanilla extract and lemon zest; gradually mix the flour mixture into the beer mixture until it becomes a smooth batter.

3. Melt the coconut oil in a skillet over medium heat. When the oil is hot, dip the quince wedges into the batter and place them in the hot oil; fry in batches until golden brown. Remove fried quinces to a warm platter while you finish frying. Sprinkle the fried quinces with demerara sugar to serve.

8. Flavorful Southern Fried Chicken

Prep Time: 20 mins

Total Time: 40 mins

Servings: 4

Ingredients

- ⅔ cup all-purpose flour
- ⅔ cup grated Parmesan cheese
- 1 ⅓ cups bread crumbs
- 1 teaspoon poultry seasoning
- ½ teaspoon onion powder
- ½ teaspoon garlic powder
- ½ teaspoon salt
- ½ teaspoon pepper
- 1 ½ cups milk
- 12 ounces chicken tenderloins
- 1 ½ cups vegetable oil for frying

Directions

1. In a large plastic bag, combine the flour, Parmesan cheese, bread crumbs, poultry seasoning, onion powder, garlic powder, salt and pepper. Shake to mix.
2. Heat the oil in a large skillet over medium heat until a drop of water evaporates immediately. Dip

one piece of chicken at a time into the milk, and then place in the bag with the coating. Shake until fully coated. Place in the frying pan, and continue with remaining chicken.

3. Cook until the edges are browned, then flip and cook until browned on the other side. If some chicken is done sooner, keep on a paper towel lined plate in a warm oven, so that the chicken is all still warm at serving time.

9. Grilled Blood Orange Chuck Steak

Prep Time: 15 mins

Total Time: 8 hrs 25 mins

Servings: 6

Ingredients

- ½ cup blood orange marmalade
- ¼ cup water
- ¼ cup soy sauce
- ¼ cup prepared mojo criollo dressing
- 2 tablespoons brown sugar
- 2 tablespoons orange juice
- 1 teaspoon ground ginger
- ¼ teaspoon garlic powder
- 1 ½ teaspoons grated orange zest
- 2 pounds beef chuck steak

Directions

1. Mix marmalade, water, soy sauce, mojo criollo dressing, brown sugar, orange juice, ginger, garlic powder, and orange zest in a bowl. Measure 1 cup marinade and pour into a large resealable plastic bag; add beef to bag. Seal bag and turn beef inside bag to coat completely. Marinate in refrigerator, turning occasionally, for at least 8 hours to

overnight. Cover bowl with remaining marinade and refrigerate.

2. Remove beef from marinade; discard used marinade.
3. Preheat grill for medium heat and lightly oil the grate.
4. Grill beef on the preheated grill, basting frequently with reserved marinade, until desired doneness is reached, 5 to 10 minutes per side. An instant-read thermometer inserted into the center should read 140 degrees F (60 degrees C).

10. Ham with Honey and Brown Sugar Glaze

Prep Time: 30 mins

Total Time: 1 hr 30 mins

Servings: 8

Ingredients

- 1 (5 pound) fully cooked sliced ham
- ¼ cup whole cloves
- 1 cup pineapple juice
- 1 cup brown sugar
- ½ cup honey
- 2 oranges, juiced

Directions

1. Preheat the oven to 350 degrees F (175 degrees C).
2. Place the ham in a roasting pan and dot with cloves. In a saucepan combine the pineapple juice, brown sugar, honey and orange juice. Stir and simmer over medium-low heat until thickened, about 10 minutes. Pour the glaze over the ham.
3. Bake the ham uncovered for 1 hour in the preheated oven.

Prep Time: 30 mins

Total Time: 1 hr 30 mins

Servings: 8

Ingredients

- 5 tablespoons all-purpose flour
- ¼ teaspoon salt
- 1 cup white sugar
- 2 ½ cups heavy whipping cream
- 1 recipe pastry for a 9 inch single crust pie
- ½ teaspoon ground cinnamon

Directions

1. Preheat oven to 375 degrees F (190 degrees C).
2. Mix flour, sugar and salt together. Add the whipping cream and mix thoroughly. Pour batter into one unbaked 9" pie shell. Sprinkle top with cinnamon.
3. Bake at 375 degrees F (190 degrees C) for 45 minutes to 60 minutes or until bubbly all over the top. Store the baked pie in the refrigerator.

12. Vegetable Soup with Quinoa

Prep Time: 25 mins

Total Time: 1 hr 15 mins

Servings: 10

Ingredients

- 3 tablespoons olive oil
- 3 medium onions, chopped
- 2 green bell peppers, chopped
- 1 carrot, diced
- 1 stalk celery, diced
- 6 cloves garlic, minced
- 3 tablespoons ground cumin
- 1 teaspoon chili powder
- 1 (28 ounce) can crushed tomatoes
- 10 green chile peppers, seeded and minced
- 8 cups vegetable broth
- 1 (15 ounce) can chickpeas, drained
- ½ cup quinoa
- salt and ground black pepper to taste
- 1 ½ cups frozen corn, thawed
- 1 avocado - peeled, pitted, and diced

Directions

1. Heat oil in a large stock pot over medium heat. Stir in onions, bell peppers, carrot, celery, garlic,

cumin, and chili powder. Cook until vegetables are tender, about 10 minutes.

2. Mix in crushed tomatoes and green chile peppers. Pour in broth, chickpeas, and quinoa. Season with salt and pepper. Bring to a boil; reduce heat to low and simmer for 30 minutes.

3. Mix corn into the soup until heated through, about 5 minutes. Serve in bowls and top with avocado.

13. Shortbread

Servings: 6

Ingredients

- ¼ cup white sugar
- ½ cup unsalted butter
- 1 cup all-purpose flour
- ⅓ cup white rice flour

Directions

1. Preheat oven to 325 degrees F (165 degrees C).
2. Line a baking sheet with greaseproof (parchment) paper. Sift the flour and rice flour into a medium mixing bowl. Add the sugar and mix.
3. Cut butter into pieces and rub into the flour with your fingertips until the mixture begins to bind together. Knead into soft dough.
4. Roll the dough into an 8 inch round (or for exact round, mold it in an 8 inch cake pan). Place on baking sheet. Using a fork, prick top and make tine marks along edge. Using a table knife, score top with wedge marks. (This is where it will break when cooled)
5. Bake 45 minutes or until pale golden in color. Sprinkle a little superfine sugar over top and cool on baking sheet.

6. Cut into wedges. Keeps for weeks in airtight tin.

29

14. Russian Green Bean and Potato Soup

Prep Time: 25 mins

Total Time: 55 mins

Servings: 6

Ingredients

- 1 tablespoon vegetable oil
- 1 large onion, halved and thinly sliced
- 4 red potatoes, cubed
- ½ pound green beans, cut into 1 inch pieces
- 5 cups vegetable, chicken, or beef broth
- 2 tablespoons whole wheat flour
- ½ cup sour cream
- ¾ cup sauerkraut with juice
- 1 tablespoon chopped fresh dill
- Salt and pepper to taste

Directions

1. Heat vegetable oil in a large saucepan over medium heat. Stir in the onion, and gently cook until softened and translucent, about 5 minutes. Add the potatoes and green beans; cook until the green beans have slightly softened, about 5 more minutes.

2. Pour in the vegetable stock. Bring to a boil over high heat, then lower heat to medium-low, cover, and cook until the potatoes have softened, about 15 minutes. Stir the flour into the sour cream, and add it a spoonful at a time to the simmering soup. Stir in the sauerkraut and dill, season to taste with salt and pepper. Simmer for 5 minutes more before serving.

15. Double Chocolate Chip Cookies

Prep ime: 15 mins

Total Time: 25 mins

Servings: 40

Ingredients

- 1 cup margarine, softened
- 1 cup white sugar
- 1 cup brown sugar
- 2 eggs
- 1 teaspoon vanilla extract
- 2 cups all-purpose flour
- 1 teaspoon baking soda
- 1 teaspoon salt
- ⅓ cup unsweetened cocoa powder
- 3 cups semisweet chocolate chips

Directions

1. Preheat the oven to 375 degrees F (190 degrees C). Grease cookie sheets.
2. In a medium bowl, cream together the margarine, white sugar, and brown sugar until smooth. Beat in the eggs one at a time, then stir in the vanilla. Sift in the flour, baking soda, salt, and cocoa powder; mix well. Stir in the chocolate chips. Roll

tablespoonfuls of cookie dough into balls and place them 1 inch apart onto the prepared cookie sheets.

3. Bake for 8 to 10 minutes in the preheated oven. Allow cookies to cool on baking sheet for 2 minutes before removing to a wire rack to cool completely.

16. Crisp Peach Cobbler

Prep Time: 20 mins

Total Time: 1 hr 35 mins

Servings: 8

Ingredients

Batter:

- ½ cup unsalted butter, at room temperature
- 1 ¼ cups white sugar
- 1 ⅓ cups self-rising flour
- ⅓ cup rolled oats
- ⅔ cup whole milk

Glaze:

- ¼ cup white sugar
- 2 tablespoons cold water, or as needed to wet topping sugar

Directions

1. Preheat oven to 375 degrees F (190 degrees C). Place a baking sheet on the rack under the middle rack to catch drips. Generously butter a 2-inch deep (2-quart) baking dish.

2. Place peach sections into prepared baking dish. Sprinkle with lemon juice and zest.

3. Stir butter and sugar together in a mixing bowl. Mix until creamed and resembles a sugary, buttery paste, 4 to 5 minutes. Add oats and flour; stir until flour and oats are incorporated into the butter-sugar mixture and mixture resembles coarse crumbs, 4 to 5 minutes. Pour in milk; stir until mixture is wet and creamy, like a thick spreadable batter, 3 to 4 minutes.

4. Drop batter by spoonful on top of the peaches. Spread batter evenly over the surface of the peaches. Sprinkle 1/4 cup sugar on the batter. Spritz with water until sugar is wet and surface glistens.

5. Bake in preheated oven on middle rack until browned and crispy, about 45 minutes. Let cool at least 30 minutes before serving.

17. Broccoli and Tomato Bake

Prep Time: 30 mins

Total Time: 1 hr 15 mins

Servings: 4

Ingredients

- 1 tablespoon olive oil
- 1 small onion, thinly sliced
- 1 clove garlic, minced
- 1 small carrot, diced
- 1 stalk celery, diced
- salt and ground black pepper
- ¾ pound broccoli - cut into florets, stems peeled and sliced 1/4 inch thick
- 1 (15 ounce) can diced tomatoes
- 1 tablespoon chopped green olives
- 2 teaspoons maple syrup
- ¼ cup crumbled goat cheese
- ¼ cup Parmesan cheese

Directions

1. Heat olive oil in a skillet over medium heat. Add the onion and garlic; cook and stir until aromatic, about 3 minutes. Stir in the carrots and celery, season with salt and pepper, and continue

cooking until the vegetables begin to soften, about 5 minutes.

Meanwhile, place a steamer insert into a saucepan, and fill with water to just below the bottom of the steamer. Cover, and bring the water to a boil over high heat. Add the broccoli, recover, and steam until bright green, 4 minutes. Remove the broccoli from the steamer and place in a 8x8 inch baking dish; set aside.

2. Preheat an oven to 375 degrees F (190 degrees C).

3. Pour the can of diced tomatoes and green olives into the skillet with the onion and carrot mixture. Stir and cook over medium-high heat until most of the sauce thickens, about 5 minutes. Mix in the maple syrup, season with salt and pepper to taste, and cook and stir for 3 minutes.

4. Pour the sauce over the broccoli in the 8x8 inch baking dish. Evenly distribute the goat cheese and Parmesan cheese over the broccoli and sauce.

5. Bake in preheated oven until the cheese begins to brown, about 20 minutes.

18. Easy Mostaccioli Pasta Salad

Prep Time: 10 mins

Total Time: 25 m

Servings: 4

Ingredients

- 1 (16 ounce) package mostaccioli pasta
- 1 cup Italian-style salad dressing
- 1 cup creamy salad dressing
- 1 tablespoon white sugar
- 1 tablespoon dried parsley
- ¼ teaspoon salt
- ¼ teaspoon ground black pepper
- ¼ teaspoon garlic salt
- ¼ teaspoon Italian seasoning
- ¼ teaspoon celery seed
- ¼ teaspoon mustard seed

Directions

1. Bring a large pot of lightly salted water to a boil. Add pasta and cook, stirring occasionally, until tender yet firm to the bite, about 11 minutes. Drain and put into a large bowl.
2. Combine Italian salad dressing, creamy salad dressing, sugar, parsley, salt, pepper, garlic salt, Italian seasoning, celery seed, and mustard seed

in a smaller bowl. Pour the dressing over the noodles and stir to combine. Refrigerate until needed.

Prep Time: 25 mins

Total Time: 2 hrs 30 mins

Servings: 14

Ingredients

Crust:

- 3 tablespoons butter
- 1 cup graham cracker crumbs
- 1 tablespoon white sugar

Filling:

- 4 eggs
- 1 cup white sugar
- 4 (8 ounce) packages cream cheese, softened
- 1 (16 ounce) package cottage cheese
- 1 teaspoon vanilla extract

Frosting:

- 1 (16 ounce) container sour cream
- ½ cup white sugar
- ½ teaspoon vanilla extract

Directions

1. Preheat the oven to 300 degrees F (150 degrees C).
2. Melt butter in a 8x2-inch round springform pan in the preheated oven. Let cool 10 minutes.
3. Combine graham cracker crumbs and sugar in a bowl; mix well. Pat mixture into the bottom of the springform pan with butter.
4. Bake crust in the preheated oven until golden and set, about 10 minutes. Remove from the oven and let cool.
5. While crust is cooling, beat eggs using an electric mixer in a bowl for 3 minutes. Add 1 cup sugar and beat for 2 minutes more. Mix in cream cheese and cottage cheese slowly, adding one package of cream cheese at a time. Pour in 1 teaspoon vanilla extract; beat for 10 minutes. Pour filling into the cooled crust.
6. Bake in the preheated oven until firmly set, about 1 hour.
7. While cake is baking, mix together sour cream, 1/2 cup sugar, and 1/2 teaspoon vanilla extract for frosting. Set aside and allow to reach room temperature.
8. Remove cheesecake from the oven. Spread frosting carefully onto the top of the warm cheesecake.
9. Return cheesecake to the oven and bake until topping is golden and set, 10 to 12 minutes more.

10. Turn off the oven and allow cake to cool to near-room temperature in the oven, as this is key in preventing cracks or dips in cake top, about 30 minutes. Remove from the oven and chill in the refrigerator until ready to serve.

20. Mama's Chewy Oatmeal Cookies

Prep Time: 15 mins

Total Time: 25 mins

Servings: 48

Ingredients

- 2 cups packed brown sugar
- 1 cup shortening
- ⅓ cup milk
- 1 egg
- 1 teaspoon vanilla extract
- 4 cups quick cooking oats
- 1 ¾ cups all-purpose flour, or more if needed
- 1 teaspoon baking soda
- 1 teaspoon salt

Directions

1. Preheat oven to 375 degrees F (190 degrees C).
2. Beat brown sugar, shortening, milk, egg, and vanilla extract in a bowl until mixture is creamy. Stir oats, flour, baking soda, and salt into moist ingredients. Drop dough by spoonful onto ungreased baking sheets.
3. Bake in the preheated oven until cookies are lightly golden brown, 8 to 10 minutes.

21. Moms Fresh Cranberry-Pumpkin Bread

Prep Time: 15 mins

Total Time: 1 hr 25 mins

Servings: 20

Ingredients

- 1 serving cooking spray
- 3 ½ cups all-purpose flour
- 2 ½ cups white sugar
- 1 ½ tablespoons pumpkin pie spice
- 2 teaspoons baking soda
- 1 ½ cups canned pumpkin puree
- 4 eggs
- ⅔ cup milk
- ½ cup canola oil
- 1 (12 ounce) package fresh cranberries

Directions

1. Preheat the oven to 325 degrees F (165 degrees C). Grease two 9x5-inch loaf pan with cooking spray.
2. Combine flour, sugar, pumpkin pie spice, and baking soda in a large bowl.
3. Combine pumpkin puree, eggs, milk, and oil in a separate bowl. Add to the dry ingredients and

beat until well combined. Add cranberries and stir to blend. Divide batter between the prepared pans.

4. Bake in the preheated oven until a toothpick inserted into the center comes out clean, about 1 hour. Cool in the pans for 10 minutes, then remove to cooling racks to cool completely.

22. Raspberry Cheesecake Stuffed French Toast

Prep Time: 20 mins

Total Time: 30 mins

Servings: 6

Ingredients

- 1 cup milk
- 2 tablespoons vanilla extract
- 1 cup white sugar
- 2 tablespoons cinnamon
- 4 eggs, beaten
- 1 cup raspberry puree
- 4 ounces cream cheese, softened
- 1 loaf French bread, cut into 1 inch slices
- butter
- confectioners' sugar for dusting
- nutmeg, for topping

Directions

1. In a bowl, whisk milk, vanilla, sugar, and cinnamon into the beaten eggs until well blended. Set aside. In a separate bowl, cream together raspberry puree and cream cheese until smooth. Make 'sandwiches' by cutting each slice of bread

in half and spreading raspberry-cheese mixture in the center, then top with the other half.

2. Melt butter over medium heat in a large skillet or griddle. Dip bread into egg mixture, coating thoroughly. Cook until well-browned on both sides, about 5 minutes. Dust with confectioners' sugar and nutmeg. Serve immediately.

23. Dutch Oven Chili Colorado

Prep Time: 30 mins

Total Time: 3 hrs 5 mins

Servings: 12

Ingredients

- 4 ancho chiles
- 4 pounds boneless beef chuck, trimmed and cut into 3/4-inch pieces
- 1 pinch salt and freshly ground black pepper to taste
- 2 medium onions, coarsely chopped
- 6 cloves garlic
- ¼ cup ground red chile pepper
- 2 teaspoons salt
- 1 teaspoon cumin seeds
- 1 teaspoon dried oregano
- ½ teaspoon ground coriander
- 1 cup Mexican beer, or more as needed

Directions

1. Soak the ancho chiles in boiling hot water to cover for 1 hour.

2. While dried chiles soak, preheat the oven to 350 degrees F (175 degrees C). Season beef with salt and pepper.

3. Heat a cast iron Dutch oven over medium-high heat. Brown the beef on all sides, working in small batches, 5 to 7 minutes. Set aside.

4. Drain chiles; remove stems and seeds. Place chiles, onions, garlic, ground chile pepper, salt, cumin seeds, oregano, and coriander in the bowl of a food processor. Pulse to chop, then process into a thick paste. Add 1 cup beer and continue processing to blend.

5. Place meat and any accumulated juices back in the Dutch oven, pour in sauce, and stir well. Cover with a sheet of aluminum foil, then place lid on top for a tight seal.

6. Bake on the middle rack of the preheated oven for 1 hour; stir. Continue to bake, stirring every 15 minutes, until meat is fork-tender, 30 minutes to 1 hour more, adding more beer if sauce seems too thick.

24. Mayo Free Cabbage Salad

Prep Time: 10 mins

Total Time: 1 hr 10 mins

Servings: 10

Ingredients

- ½ cup canola oil
- ¼ cup red wine vinegar
- 1 tablespoon soy sauce
- 6 tablespoons white sugar
- 1 (8 ounce) package shredded cabbage
- 3 green onions, thinly sliced
- ⅓ cup slivered almonds
- ⅓ cup sunflower seed kernels

Directions

1. Mix canola oil, red wine vinegar, soy sauce, and sugar in a large bowl, mixing until sugar has dissolved. Toss cabbage, green onions, almonds, and sunflower seed kernels into the dressing. Cover bowl and refrig

Prep Time: 25 mins

Total Time: 45 mins

Servings: 4

Ingredients

- 1 (8 ounce) package cavatelli pasta
- 1 head broccoli, cut into florets
- ½ cup butter
- 3 cloves garlic, finely chopped
- 1 (4.5 ounce) can sliced mushrooms, drained
- ¼ cup grated Parmesan cheese

Directions

2. Preheat oven to 350 degrees F (175 degrees C).
3. Bring a large pot of lightly salted water to a boil. Add pasta and cook for 8 to 10 minutes or until al dente; drain.
4. Place broccoli in a microwave safe dish with about 3 tablespoons of water. Microwave for 3 minutes, or until tender.
5. Melt butter in a medium skillet over medium heat. Saute garlic and mushrooms until garlic becomes aromatic. Combine with pasta, broccoli

and Parmesan cheese; transfer to a 2 quart baking dish.
6. Cover and bake in preheated oven for about 20 minutes, or until heated throughout

26. Swiss Steak

Prep Time: 15 mins

Total Time: 2 hrs

Servings: 6

Ingredients

- ¼ cup all-purpose flour
- ½ teaspoon salt
- ¼ teaspoon ground black pepper
- 1 (2 pound) beef round steak, 1 inch thick
- 2 tablespoons vegetable shortening
- ¼ cup water, or as needed
- 1 (8 ounce) can diced tomatoes
- 1 onion, minced
- ½ green bell pepper, chopped
- salt and ground black pepper to taste

Directions

1. Mix flour, 1/2 teaspoon salt, and 1/4 teaspoon black pepper together in a bowl. Sprinkle half the flour mixture on one side of round steak pieces; pound steak until coating is absorbed. Flip steak and coat with remaining flour mixture; pound steak until coating is absorbed. Cut steak into 6 pieces.

2. Melt shortening in a large skillet over medium heat; place steak pieces in the hot shortening. Cook until browned, 7 to 10 minutes per side. Cover and simmer until tender, about 1 hour, adding water as needed.
3. Turn steak pieces over and add tomatoes, onion, and green bell pepper to the skillet. Season with salt and black pepper. Simmer until vegetables are tender, about 30 more minutes.

27. Traditional Sauerbraten

Prep Time: 15 mins

Total Time: 2 days 4 hrs 15 mins

Servings: 6

Ingredients

- 3 pounds beef rump roast
- 2 large onions, chopped
- 1 cup red wine vinegar, or to taste
- 1 cup water
- 1 tablespoon salt
- 1 tablespoon ground black pepper
- 1 tablespoon white sugar
- 10 whole cloves, or more to taste
- 2 bay leaves, or more to taste
- 2 tablespoons all-purpose flour
- salt and ground black pepper to taste
- 2 tablespoons vegetable oil
- 10 gingersnap cookies, crumbled

Directions

1. Place beef rump roast, onions, vinegar, water, 1 tablespoon salt, 1 tablespoon black pepper, sugar, cloves, and bay leaves in a large pot. Cover and refrigerate for 2 to 3 days, turning meat daily.

Remove meat from marinade and pat dry with paper towels, reserving marinade.

2. Season flour to taste with salt and black pepper in a large bowl. Sprinkle flour mixture over beef.
3. Heat vegetable oil in a large Dutch oven or pot over medium heat; cook beef until brown on all sides, about 10 minutes. Pour reserved marinade over beef, cover, and reduce heat to medium-low. Simmer until beef is tender, 3 1/2 to 4 hours. Remove beef to a platter and slice.
4. Strain solids from remaining liquid and continue cooking over medium heat. Add gingersnap cookies and simmer until gravy is thickened, about 10 minutes. Serve gravy over sliced beef.

28. Fried Cabbage with Bacon and Garlic

Prep Time: 15 mins

Total Time: 40 mins

Servings: 6

Ingredients

- 1 (1 pound) package bacon, finely chopped
- 1 teaspoon olive oil
- 1 medium onion, chopped
- 2 cloves garlic, minced
- 2 pounds diced cabbage
- ½ teaspoon salt
- ½ teaspoon ground black pepper
- ¼ teaspoon red pepper flakes

Directions

1. Place bacon in a large skillet and cook over medium-high heat, stirring occasionally, until browned and crispy, 7 to 10 minutes. Drain bacon slices on paper towels and remove most of the bacon grease from the skillet.
2. Add oil to the skillet and heat over medium heat. Add onion and garlic; cook and stir until the onion has softened and turned translucent, about 5 minutes. Add cabbage, salt, pepper, and red

pepper flakes; cook and stir until cabbage is tender, 10 to 15 minutes. If you prefer softer cabbage, cover the skillet while cooking to give it some steam.

3. Crumble bacon into the skillet and mix with the cabbage until well combine

Prep Time: 40 mins

Total Time: 1 hr 10 mins

Servings: 45

Ingredients

- 18 ½ ounces extra sharp Cheddar cheese, shredded
- ½ cup butter, softened
- ½ teaspoon paprika
- 1 ½ cups all-purpose flour
- 45 pitted green olives

Directions

1. Allow cheese to sit out until it is at room temperature. In a large bowl, mix together the cheese, butter and paprika using a pastry blender. Gradually mix in flour, first using the pastry blender, then using your hands. Mix until the dough pulls together. It should form a solid ball with a smooth appearance, but have a crumbly texture when pulled apart. If dough appears too dry, add more shredded cheese.
2. Preheat the oven to 375 degrees F (190 degrees C). Pinch off a small piece of dough, and cover an

olive with it. Roll gently between your palms to smooth and seal the olive inside the ball. Place onto an ungreased cookie sheet and repeat with remaining dough and olives. Place the tray of covered olives into the refrigerator for 10 minutes to firm up.

3. Bake for 20 to 25 minutes in the preheated oven, or until browned. Serve hot or at room temperature.

30. Holiday Goat Cheese Log

Prep Time: 15 mins

Total Time: 15 mins

Servings: 8

Ingredients

- ½ cup smoked almonds
- 2 tablespoons roughly chopped fresh parsley
- 2 tablespoons roughly chopped fresh chives
- ¼ cup dried cherries
- 1 (8 ounce) log plain goat cheese

Directions

1. Pulse almonds in the bowl of a food processor until chopped. Add parsley and chives; continue to pulse until incorporated. Add cherries and process until everything is finely chopped and you have a nice mixture of red and green.
2. Pour nut mixture onto a flat work surface and spread into a thin layer.
3. Roll goat cheese log in the nut mixture until fully covered. Carefully pick it up and tap the ends of the log into the nut mixture to cover. Place on a serving dish.